The Essential Art of Aromatherapy

Rebecca Nicely

ISBN: 978-1537607108
ISBN-13: 1537607103

The FDA has not evaluated the statements in this book or on my website. No claims are made as to any medicinal value of these tips, formulas, products or suggestions. Products, information, and descriptions presented here are for educational purposes of the traditional uses of essential oils and herbs only and are not intended to diagnose, treat, cure, or prevent any disease. This information should not be used as a substitute for medical counseling with a health care professional. Individuals who are under a physicians care for any condition, including pregnancy or nursing, should consult a qualified health care professional prior to using any of the remedies in this book.

Essential oils are very highly concentrated and potent and it is important to always check the specific safety data provided from the manufacturer. Keep out of reach of children, the elderly and pets. For external use only. Avoid contact with mucus membranes and eyes. If any essential oils have contacted your eye, wash out with a vegetable oil such as olive oil, not water, and seek medical attention immediately.

Some oils may cause skin irritation in people with sensitive skin. It is recommended to perform a patch test before use. To patch test, place one drop on the back of your wrist and leave for an hour or more. If irritation or redness occurs, wash the area with olive oil followed by cold water. Discontinue use of that oil. Consult a physician if irritation persists. I do not recommend the ingestion of essential oils.

DEDICATION

For all before me who blazed the path, those
who walk with me in love and to those whose
greatness has yet to be revealed.
Live in light and shine on!

CONTENTS

ACKNOWLEDGMENTS

In the winding journey of my life, I have many things to be grateful for. Most of all, I am thankful for the moments. The simple things: a well timed hug, a shared cup of tea, a slow smile, grass under my feet. May I always be fully present to acknowledge these gifts. And above all, I'd like to thank my soul family for your love, constant support and inspiration.

1

WHERE DO I BEGIN?

Begin where you are right now. This little book has no expectations. Whew, right? So many aromatherapy guides leave you feeling like you have to have tons of prior knowledge on multiple subjects, expensive rare ingredients on hand and many throw around Latin and Sanskrit like they're ordering a drink at the coffee shop. I have good news! Not this one. We're going to start slowly and simply, with items you probably already have in your pantry. My intention is to offer a guidebook that is full of simple, honest to goodness tips that have worked for me, my family and my friends for many years.

As in life, not everything will work for everyone. Some things might not resonate now, but will down the road. I've learned to trust the process. Is something happening in your life that you need a little support? Turn right to that chapter. I do encourage you to go back and read the entire book when things settle down. My guess is, once you've read a little, you're going to want to anyway.

If you're new to this kind of thing, please go ahead and read straight through. I've organized it in a way that you won't be overwhelmed. In light of keeping this a small guide, we'll touch on a few topics more than others. For those that peak your interest, follow your curiosity and see where it takes you in further research. I'll include resources at the end of the book that I found helped on my journey.

I encourage you to make notes in the margins, take out your markers and underline things, pull out some washi tape and make bookmarks. It's your book and meant to be a guide on your new adventure. Please make it your own. That's when the magic happens.

As you go through the pages, please feel free to reach out to me with questions and comments. I love nothing more than to hear how a seemly simple tip has changed someone's life. In fact, it happens almost every day.

Now, let's take a deep breath and go exploring!

2

WHAT IS AROMATHERAPY?

So, let's get down to business and talk a little bit about the aromatherapy. We're going to define all the important players in this amazing art. I promise, it's not going to be boring. Just enough for you to know what you need to know before we jump in deeper.

Aromatherapy is the art of using plant derived, aromatic essential oils for therapeutic purposes to promote physical and psychological well being. Yep, that's a lot to take in, so let's break it down.

What are essential oils? They are the volatile concentrated liquids that are extracted from the leaves, stems, flowers, roots or bark of a plant. Essential Oils are generally seventy times more concentrated than whole plants. All these essential oils are grouped based on the effects they create in the body. You will hear them referred to as cooling, warming, calming, energizing or stimulating. Beyond that, many are valued more medicinally, as anti septic and anti viral.

The majority of essential oils are obtained through distillation, with the exception being citrus oils, which are extracted through cold pressing. I won't get into the details, but it's an intensive process that gives us few precious drops of these highly concentrated, amazing essential oils. You're probably wondering, how concentrated are they, really? It takes approximately 200 pounds of lavender flowers to make 1 pound of lavender essential oil. To create one 10 ml bottle of Lemon Essential Oil, 70 lemons need to be cold pressed. Most essential oils are clear, except for some of the citruses and woodsier oils, which vary from golden to brown.

Now that you know what they are, you're probably wondering just how to use them? For our purposes, we're going to concentrate on two ways to incorporate aromatherapy into your life: inhalation and application to the skin.

The most commonly used method of aromatherapy is though inhalation. Airborne essential oil molecules are inhaled through the nose, interact with the olfactory organs and effect the brain almost immediately through a variety of systems and key receptor areas. One of the most notable is the limbic system response. The limbic system is a pathway to the parts of the brain that control breathing, stress levels, memory, blood pressure and hormone balance. When aromatherapy is used, we can assist with imbalances. Did you ever wonder why the scent of vanilla takes you right back to your grandma's cozy kitchen? Now you know.

The benefits of aromatherapy are also seen when essential oils are inhaled through the mouth. The essential oil molecules are carried to the lungs and interact with the respiratory system. This is often why eucalyptus is inhaled to help with a cough. In the next chapter, we'll learn about tools for diffusing aromatherapy in the air.

3

WHAT'S A DIFFUSER, ANYWAY?

It's time to replace those artificial air fresheners with some beautiful aromatherapy! The easiest way to receive immediate benefits and make your home smell amazing, is through the use of a diffuser.

There are four basic types of diffusers: nebulizers, ultrasonic, heat and evaporative. All of them have their benefits. I'll talk a bit about their qualities so you can decide which one is perfect for you.

Aromatherapists create essential oil blends for use in diffusers or other methods for inhalation. At it's most basic, a diffuser is just a vehicle to get the aromatherapy into the air, so you can inhale it. There are many types of diffusers available today.

My favorite everyday diffusers are Ultrasonic Diffusers. You add a few drops of essential oils to water and the diffuser creates a cool, fine mist. They are affordable and easy to take care of. I have not found any tea light burner, heat diffuser or clay diffuser that compare.

The next tool you can use is a nebulizing diffuser. Nebulizing diffusers put the whole drop of pure essential oils directly into the air from an attached bottle. Nebulizer diffusers are truly works of art to me. They work a lot like a perfume atomizer. The top portion is usually made of a hand blown pyrex glass, which is attached to a bottle of essential oils. They are very powerful and offer a continuous stream of concentrated aromatherapy. Because of that, they do use oils quickly and they can be pricey. They do not need heat or water to operate. I use these for professional aromatherapy treatments and when there is need to get aromatherapy into the air quickly. I recommend using a timer with your nebulizer and using for fifteen minutes at a time.

Tea light candle burners can also be used. You fill the top bowl with water and a few drops of essential oils and then light the tea light candle below to heat the oils. This disperses the oils into the air. There are two main issues with using these type of diffusers: the water will boil off, so you need to keep a close eye on your burner and heated essential oils lose a bit of their therapeutic benefit as the composition of the essential oil is changed when heat is applied.

Evaporative diffusers use a fan to blow air through a pad that has essential oils applied to it. The stream of air causes the oils to be blown into the room and evaporate at a quicker rate than usual. This process tends to break down the oils into separate components, instead of getting the whole oil at once. The lighter parts at at the beginning of the diffusion process, followed by the heavier components toward the end. These diffusers do have positive points, though. You can fill a room quickly with aromatherapy and they're pretty quiet to run.

A new trend is aromatherapy jewelry. Beautiful unfired clay pieces, carved wood and natural lava rocks are being used to make jewelry little pendant and beads so you can take aromatherapy with you. You just apply a drop or two of essential oils, let it dry and wear throughout the day to experience the light scent of your blend. There are also pretty clay medallions that you can add oils to and place throughout your home for aromatherapy in closets, storage and other places more complex diffusers wouldn't be feasible.

The last main diffusers are heat diffusers, which simply use heat to disperse the essential oils into the air. A common type is an auto diffuser that plugs into the cigarette lighter. You place a few drops of essential oils on a cotton pad, then put the pad on a metal plate in the diffuser. The whole thing plugs in and soon your car fills with your favorite blend. There also are a few companies that make in home heat diffusers that look like flying saucers. They can work like the auto diffuser with a cotton pad and metal plate or they may just have a small metal bowl that you add essential oils to. Again, the issue with this type is the heat can change the makeup of the essential oils, making your experience less therapeutic.

4

YOUR SKIN IS YOUR LARGEST ORGAN

Did you ever think about what happens to all those products you apply to your skin? Most of them end up in your bloodstream. Crazy, right? So it makes sense that aromatherapy works well through topical application. Consider your skin for a moment. It is permeable, which makes it a perfect pathway for essential oils. Due to their small molecular size, they penetrate the skin easily and enter the bloodstream. And because essential oils are so concentrated, a little goes a long way.

In most cases essential oils need to be mixed with a neutral oil, called a carrier. A carrier is most typically a type of oil that blends with the essential oils to make them safe to apply to the skin. Common carrier oils include: sweet almond oil, coconut oil, jojoba and hemp seed oil.

Another popular way of applying essential oils to the skin is by adding the essential oils to a pre-made base. You can add them to any organic unscented shower gel, body lotion or massage oil and make your own blends. Please make sure the base you use is organic, as we want to ensure the essential oils can work their magic without any nasty chemicals getting in the way.

When applying essential oils to the skin using a carrier oil or another base, it is very important to understand how to dilute the essential oils properly for the maximum therapeutic benefit. We will discuss dilution in more detail in a later chapter.

5

HOW TO CHOOSE
THE BEST OILS

If you do an internet search for essential oils you'll find tens of thousands of results. Due to the popularity of aromatherapy, there has been a huge surge in essential oil offerings. This can be quite overwhelming, but you have come to the right place. I'm going to give you some tips to make it as easy as possible to start using high quality, therapeutic oils.

Now that we know how aromatherapy works, it's very important to use essential oils that are as pure as possible. For example, if we are trying to ease headache pain that may be caused by toxins, we would never want to use essential oils that have been stretched with the addition of synthetic chemicals. When your body uptakes these modified oils, the therapeutic benefit of the aromatherapy is lost and you're adding to your troubles by introducing more chemicals into the mix. Since we know now that all the essential oils we use are either assimilate through our olfactory system or absorption through our skin, I believe we should treat them like we would our food.

And remember, there is a big difference in the amount of essential oils obtained from different plants. This is reflected in the wide ranging prices of essential oils. Lemons have a relatively high yield and therefore lemon essential oil is much less expensive than rose essential oil, which uses a large quantity of rose petals to produce.   If you notice a company that sells all of their oils for the same price, there's probably something not right with the quality of the oil.

If possible, try to find essential oils that are wild crafted. Wild crafting is a process where the plants are preserved as much as possible during harvest, instead of just clear cutting them down. This leads to higher quality, heirloom oils. Look for independent testing and certifications, too.

All in all, I believe in quality over quantity. I make it a point to use organic essential oils whenever possible. Many companies have harvested the plants and created essential oils for generations.

If you have an experienced aromatherapist in your area, they are a tremendous resource for quality oils. They are in the business of using aromatherapy to help people and will be able to offer a lot of advice.

Don't be overwhelmed. A little research will lead you to wonderful essential oils. I will also include some of my favorites in the Resources section at the end of this book.

Because essential oils are plant matter, they do need some special care. They should be stored in tinted glass bottles and kept from direct sunlight and heat to maintain their medicinal benefit and to keep them from evaporating. They also will degrade over time.

For beginning purposes, it is not necessary or advised to purchase fifty big bottles of oils. You can start with a few key oils and add from there. I know what you're thinking. Which oils should I start with? Well, read on.

6

KEY ESSENTIAL OILS

As an aromatherapist, the question I'm most often asked is what oils are the best to keep on hand. I've narrowed down the vast amount of oils available to a few key essential oils to help you create a beginner kit. You'll find you'll use some more than others. Year after year I continue to return to my tried and true workhorses. I suggest starting small with just a handful of essential oils, so you can become very comfortable with each oil. Then you can add as you need a different oil for a new blend.

I'll list each essential oil and then we will delve into their particular facts. And also, as promised, there's not going to be a lot of Latin, but I'll include their botanical names in the individual profiles, as there are many different types of each oil.

Lavender Essential Oil
(Lavender angustifolia)

Parts of Plant: Flowers
Method of Extraction: Steam Distillation
Note Classification: Middle Note
Blends Well With:
Bergamot, Cedarwood, Chamomile, Clary Sage, Eucalyptus, Geranium, Lemon, Peppermint, Rosemary, Tea Tree, and many others.

I'm sure you've heard that lavender is wonderful for relaxation. A few whiffs and you'll feel stress starting to ease. Apply throughout the day to create your personal oasis.

Lavender Essential Oil has amazing skin healing properties. A drop on a bug bite will help stop itching. Apply to burns to stop pain and speed healing. A few drops applied to dry skin or eczema will help soften skin.

Looking to sleep tight? Put a few drops in your palm and take a deep breath. Inhale and exhale a few times to even out breathing. Apply to temples, wrists and bottoms of feet and you'll be off to dreamland.

If you only ever use one essential oil, make it Lavender! It is simply amazing. I carry a bottle in my purse all the time.

Roman Chamomile Essential Oil
(arthemis nobilis) and
German Chamomile Essential Oil
(matricaria chamomilla)

Parts of Plant: Flowers
Method of Extraction: Steam Distillation
Note Classification: Middle Note
Blends Well With:
Bergamot, Clary Sage, Eucalyptus, Geranium, Jasmine, Lavender, Lemon, Neroli, Rose, Tea Tree and many others.

As with most essential oils, there are different oils with the same basic name. The two main Chamomile Essential Oils are Roman Chamomile and German Chamomile. They are quite similar in their qualities, each have distinctive benefits.

German Blue Chamomile has a high azulene content, which not only gives the oil a beautiful blue color, it is very anti inflammatory. It is very often used in skin care products.

Roman Chamomile has a light apple aroma. It is primarily used for aromatherapy and for body care products, as it helps to calm.

Chamomile is a member of the Ragweed family, so should be avoided if someone has a direct allergy to Ragweed.

Lemon Essential Oil
(citrus limon)

Parts of Plant: Lemon Peel
Method of Extraction: Cold Pressed
Note Classification: Top Note
Blends Well With:
Chamomile, Eucalyptus, Frankincense, Geranium, Juniper, Lavender, Sandalwood, Ylang Ylang, and many others.

Lemon Essential Oil is powerfully cleansing and purifying. Lemon has natural antiviral, antihistamine and antibacterial properties. When diffused, lemon is very energizing and uplifting and has shown to help improve mind, body and spirit.

Approximately one thousand lemons are needed to produce one pound of lemon essential oil.

Limonene is the chemical compound that comprises the majority of lemon essential oil. It give lemon essential oil it's refreshing citrus scent.

I add ten drops of lemon essential oil to my homemade cleaning products to add a fresh smell without nasty chemicals.

It is particularly important to never use lemon essential oil without diluting it first in a carrier oil, as it can be very irritating to skin. Studies have also found that lemon essential oil is one of a few oils that promotes photosensitivity, which is sensitivity to the sun. If applied and then exposed to sunshine, sunburn and darkening of the skin may occur.

As with any essential oil, people with sensitivities should patch test lemon essential oil before applying over a wide area. Reactions vary from person to person and may change depending on the brand and strength of essential oil used. Always proceed with caution. Pregnant and nursing women and children should consult a physician before applying lemon essential oil.

Eucalyptus Essential Oil
(eucalyptus radiata)

Parts of Plant: Leaves and Twigs
Extraction Method: Steam Distillation
Note Classification: Top Note
Blends Well With:
Cedarwood, Chamomile, Geranium, Ginger,
Juniper, Lavender, Lemon, Peppermint,
Rosemary and many others.

Eucalyptus Essential Oil is one of the most
purifying and cleansing essential oils. It helps
strengthen the immune system, has anti
inflammatory, antibacterial, decongesting,
antiseptic properties as well as other medicinal
qualities. That's the reason it's commonly used
in blends to provide relief from cold and flu
symptoms.

Eucalyptus Essential Oil has also been shown
to help with dandruff and itchy scalp. Just a
few drops of Eucalyptus Oil mixes with some
coconut oil will nourish your scalp and gives
your hair a nice shine.

A quick way to freshen a room is to diffuse a
few drops of eucalyptus essential oil in your
diffuser. Add a drop or two of lemon essential
oil and you'll have a fresh smelling home in no
time.

Because it is so active, Eucalyptus should never

be ingested. Consuming large quantities may be toxic.

Geranium Essential Oil
(pelargonium graveolens)

Parts of Plant: Flowers and Leaves
Method of Extraction: Steam Distillation
Note Classification: Middle Note
Blends Well With:
Bergamot, Cedarwood, Chamomile, Clary Sage,
Jasmine, Juniper, Lemon, Patchouli,
Peppermint, Rose, Rosemary, Sandalwood,
Ylang Ylang and many others.

Throughout history, Geranium Essential Oil
has been known as a powerful healer of
circulatory problems and skin disorders. It is
also useful to heal cuts and bruises and is an
insect repellent.

One of the biggest benefits we receive from
Geranium Essential Oil is that helps balance
emotions, particularly during the challenging
times of PMS and menopause.

As if all that isn't enough, Geranium has an
amazing ability to uplift spirits and helps with
anxiety and depression. Add to a massage oil
base and massage over the body to create a
sense of calm and wellbeing.

If it's that time of the month and you're
experiencing hormonal issues, try adding a
blend of a few drops of geranium and clary sage
to your diffuser to take the edge off.

Tea Tree Essential Oil
(melaleuca alternifolia)

Parts of Plant: Leaves and Twigs
Method of Extraction: Steam Distillation
Note Classification: Middle Note
Blends Well With:
Bergamot, German Chamomile, Clary Sage,
Eucalyptus, Geranium, Juniper, Lavender,
Lemon, Peppermint, Rosemary, Ylang Ylang
and many others.

I believe everyone should always have two
bottles of essential oils with them at all times,
or at least readily handy. Tea Tree and
Lavender Essential Oils. They have so many
amazing qualities that I keep them close at
hand. Tea Tree essential oil is best known for
purifying benefits and it's ability to boost the
immune system and fight infections. It is also
known for its cleansing abilities. That's a lot of
goodness in a bottle of oil!

Tea Tree Essential Oil works to heal cuts, burns
and skin conditions like Athlete's Foot and
dandruff. It helps soothe respiratory
conditions and achy muscles. I could write a
whole book just on the benefits of Tea Tree
Essential Oil.

As I've mentioned before, I don't recommend
using any essential oils internally, especially
Tea Tree Essential Oil. It is not toxic, but you

should use special care around the eyes and nose areas. Please seek professional help for serious cuts and burns.

Peppermint Essential Oil
(mentha piperita)

Parts of Plant: Whole Plant
Method of Extraction: Steam Distillation
Note Classification: Top Note
Blends Well With:
Cypress, Eucalyptus, Frankincense, Geranium, Grapefruit, Juniper, Lavender, Lemon, Rosemary, Tea Tree, Sandalwood and many others.

Peppermint has been a very popular herbal and essential oil since ancient times. It's invigorating, helps to increase mental clarity and promotes healthy respiratory function.

It take almost 260 pounds of peppermint leaf to make one pound of peppermint essential oil. One drop of peppermint essential oil is like drinking 27 cups of peppermint tea.

Peppermint Essential Oil is one of my favorite essential oils to diffuse because it is a quick pick me up. It's cooling and refreshing it almost immediately makes a room feel perkier.

Peppermint Essential Oil also works wonders for nausea and headaches. I use it on my feet for an upset stomach and apply to my neck and temples for tension headaches.

Since Peppermint Essential Oil is very cooling

and soothing, it is amazing for sunburns and minor skin irritations. Add a few drops of Peppermint and Lavender Essential Oils to a spray bottle with apple cider vinegar and it will take the sting out of sunburn.

Peppermint Essential Oil has a high menthol component that can be bothersome to some people, even though it is non toxic. Be mindful when using it around people with sensitivity. It should also be kept away from the eye area, as it can be irritating. Please keep it away from small children and pets.

Bergamot Essential Oil
(citrus bergamia)

Part of Plant: Peel
Method of Extraction: Cold Pressed
Note Classification: Top Note
Blends Well With:
Chamomile, Clary Sage, Cypress, Frankincense, Geranium, Jasmine, Lavender, Lemon, Neroli, Orange, Rosemary, Ylang Ylang and many others.

Bergamot Essential Oil is a citrus essential oil from the Citrus Bergamia tree, which is now usually found in Italy. It is one of the most popular essential oils. Bergamot may be a familiar scent, because it's often used in perfumes and is the characteristic flavor of Earl Grey Tea.

Bergamot is bright and sunny and is used to ease depression, anxiety, stress and even skin conditions like eczema and psoriasis.

Diffuse a few drops in your diffuser to lift your spirits and calm your mind. Add it to bath soak or blend it with massage oil to help rebalance during stressful times.

As with all but a select few oils, Bergamot Essential Oil should always be diluted with a carrier oil, as it can be a skin irritant. It is best to stay out of the sun when using this oil.

Cedarwood Essential Oil
(Juniperus Virginiana)

Part of Plant: Wood Pieces
Method of Extraction: Steam Distillation
Note Classification: Base Note
Blends Well With: Bergamot, Chamomile, Cypress, Cinnamon, Frankincense, Juniper, Jasmine, Lemon, Lavender, Rose, Neroli, Rosemary and many others.

Cedarwood Essential Oil is a woody scented oil that is primarily from the Junipers Virginiana tree in North America. Its botanical name is sometimes dependent on the regions where it is found (ex. Cedars Atlantica) but the different names do not affect the medicinal uses of the oil.

It is one of the oldest essential oils, dating back to the ancient Egyptians. They used it to make incense to fragrance the air and in embalming process.

Cedarwood Essential Oil is most often used as a calming oil to relieve anxiety and stress. It offers a spiritual lift. It also helps with respiratory issues and skin problems.

A few drops of Cedarwood Essential Oil in a diffuser will drive away mosquitoes, flies and other irritating bugs.

Cedarwood Essential Oil can be irritating to the skin in a highly concentrated state. Be mindful and ensure proper dilution when using. Please never use Cedarwood Essential Oil during pregnancy.

Patchouli Essential Oil
(pogostemon cablin)

Part of Plant: Leaves
Method of Extraction: Steam Distillation
Note Classification: Base Note
Blends Well With:
Bergamot, Cedarwood, Cypress, Geranium, Grapefruit, Lavender, Neroli, Orange, Rose, Sandalwood, Vetiver and many others.

Whenever Patchouli is mentioned, most people immediately think of the 1960s, when Patchouli Essential Oil became a staple with earthy types. It was famous for being a fragrant deodorant.

Unfortunately, since it was so widely used in synthetic perfumes, Patchouli has become very polarizing. People seem to either love it or hate it. I find if I introduce people to a pure Patchouli Essential Oil without mentioning the name, most of the time it's well liked.

As an aromatherapist, I rely on Patchouli for it's beautiful skin loving properties. It's wonderful added to a carrier oil to keep skin supple and soft, reducing the appearance of fine lines and scarring.

It is also used quite often in soothing diffusion blends. I blend it into a meditation blend that I diffuse daily.

Patchouli Essential Oil is a highly concentrated, thick essential oil. Therefore, you should only use Patchouli in small doses given its strength. It can easily overpower other essential oils. If you are one of the dislikers, please give Patchouli Essential Oil another try. You may find that you really like it!

Rose Essential Oil
(rosa damascena)

Part of Plant: Flower
Method of Extraction: Steam Distilled
Note Classification: Middle Note
Blends Well With:
Bergamot, Cedarwood, Clary Sage, Geranium, Jasmine, Lavender, Lemon, Sweet Orange, Sandalwood, Ylang Ylang and many others.

For many centuries, roses have been prized for their beautiful scent. They uplift and create a calm, soothing atmosphere. They are also some of the first plants to be distilled for their essential oils.

Rose Essential Oil is extracted, using a very delicate process, from fresh rose petals. Due to the number of rose blossoms necessary for the distillation process, Rose Essential Oil is pricier than most essential oils.

It takes about sixty thousand pounds of rose petals to produce a one ounce bottle of Rose Essential Oil.

There are two primary types of oil produced from roses: rose otto and rose absolute oil. Both Rose Oils are used for the same purposes. Rose Otto is extracted through steam distillation and Rose Absolute Oil is extracted using a solvent. Rose Otto is more expensive, but many aromatherapists prefer to use it over Rose Absolute due to the chemical solvents involved. However, Rose Absolute generally has a more intense rose aroma. For our purposes, Rose Absolute is a beautiful oil and is what I'd recommend for our beginning blends.

Rose oil is a powerful essential oil, especially for women. It helps with depression, circulation, heart problems, anxiety, asthma and respiratory conditions. Rose Essential Oil is also beautiful for use on the skin.

For soft skin, add a few drops of Rose Essential Oil to a carrier oil and massage into your skin before bed. Not only will you have beautiful skin, the scent of rose blossoms will help you drift off to sleep.

A small amount of Rose Oil can help relieve headaches, but too much can do the opposite.

Ylang Ylang Essential Oil
(cananga odorata)

Part of Plant: Flowers
Method of Extraction: Steam Distillation
Note Classification: Top Note
Blends Well With:
Bergamot, Cedarwood, Geranium, Grapefruit,
Lavender, Jasmine, Neroli, Peppermint,
Sandalwood, Vetiver and many others.

Ylang Ylang Essential Oil has a beautifully
strong floral scent. It's sweet aroma is used as
a stress reducer and even an aphrodisiac.
Ylang Ylang trees are found in rain forests and
the essential oil has just recently become
widely known.

Ylang Ylang is known for its calming properties
and is a wonderful antidepressant. It helps
soothe headaches, help with skin issues, upset
stomach and assist high blood pressure.

Add a few drops to your diffuser or blend with
a carrier oil for massage to ease the stresses of
the day.

Due to its strength, Ylang Ylang can cause
headaches and nausea with improper dilution.

Rosemary Essential Oil
(rosmarinus officinalis)

Parts of Plant: Whole Plant
Method of Extraction: Steam Distillation
Note Classification: Middle Note
Blends Well With:
Bergamot, Cedarwood, Cinnamon, Clary Sage, Eucalyptus, Frankincense, Geranium, Lavender, Lemon, Peppermint, Pine, Tea Tree and many others.

Rosemary Essential Oil is wonderful to lift the dreaded brain fog. It is an amazing stimulant for the mind.   Rosemary Essential Oil also has antidepressant properties, making it amazing for memory enhancement and focus. It works well as an analgesic to soothe aching muscles, including headaches and migraines.
Rosemary has been known to be a sacred herb throughout history.

Add a few drops to your diffuser to help with memory and to relieve congestion.

A massage oil with a few drops of Rosemary Essential Oil will help with sore muscles.

Rosemary Essential Oil should be avoided if you have been diagnosed with high blood pressure or epilepsy. Please avoid during pregnancy as well

Sweet Orange Essential Oil
(citrus sinensis)

Parts of Plant: Orange Rinds
Extraction Method: Cold Pressed/Expression
Note Classification: Top Note
Blends Well With:
Bergamot, Cinnamon, Clary Sage, Eucalyptus, Frankincense, Geranium, Ginger, Juniper, Lavender, Lemon, Neroli, Patchouli, Rose, Sandalwood, Vanilla, Ylang Ylang and many others.

Sweet Orange Essential Oil is one of my favorites. It has such a light, fresh scent. It's uplifting, energizing and just plain old happy! I use it in my diffuser to clear the air, both literally and figuratively. It uplifts the mind and body while purifying the air.

Add Sweet Orange Essential Oil to a lotion base for an energizing treat throughout the day.

Frankincense Essential Oil
(Boswellia Carteri)

Part of Plant: Resin
Method of Extraction: Steam Distillation
Note Classification: Base Note
Blend Well With:
Bergamot, Cinnamon, Cypress, Geranium, Grapefruit, Lavender, Lemon, Neroli, Sweet Orange, Patchouli, Pine, Rose, Sandalwood, Vetiver, Ylang Ylang and many others.

As you can see, Frankincense Essential Oil is an oil that adds a beautiful base note to many other essential oils. It has a deep, fresh, woodsy scent.

Frankincense has been used throughout history as an incense. Frankincense was so prized, it was given as a famous gift by one of the Wise Men. It is still popular in many religious ceremonies.

Frankincense was found in King Tutankhamen's tomb, which proves that it has been valued and used for quite some time! Due to it's long history, Frankincense is known by many names: Frankincense, Olibanum and Boswellia.

Frankincense is wonderful for skin. Add a few drops to your moisturizer for added radiance.

Blend Frankincense in a carrier oil and put in a roll on bottle. Apply to pulse points throughout the day for a balancing, grounding fragrance.

Sandalwood Essential Oil
(Santalum Album)

Part of Plant: Heartwood and Roots
Method of Extraction: Steam Distillation
Note Classification: Base Note
Blends Well With: Bergamot,
Cypress, Frankincense, Lavender, Lemon,
Neroli, Sweet Orange, Patchouli, Rose, Vetiver,
Ylang Ylang and many others.

Sandalwood Essential Oil is from an evergreen, so it has an earthy and woody scent. The Essential Oil is derived from the heart of the Sandalwood tree and has been prized for over four thousand years in India.

It's best to extract Sandalwood Essential Oil from a mature tree, which can take years. This is one of the reasons you'll notice that Sandalwood essential oil is more expensive than other essential oils. The other big reason is that over harvesting had made Sandalwood almost extinct. The good news is, Australian Sandalwood is being produced in a environmentally responsible and sustainable way, so we will not lose this amazing oil.

Sandalwood Essential Oil is used most often for relaxation and grounding in essential oil blends and perfumes. Sandalwood Essential Oil is beloved as a sacred, spiritual oil around the world and is widely used to enhance meditation and prayer. Sandalwood helps calm a busy mind.

Sandalwood Essential Oil is very hydrating and anti inflammatory, which makes it perfect for promoting healthy, smooth skin. If you experience issues with dry, chapped skin, a few drops of Sandalwood Essential Oil will help restore balance.

Mix a few drops in a carrier oil and apply to the middle of your forehead before your meditation and prayer time to experience the beauty of Sandalwood Essential Oil.

7

THE ART OF BLENDING

So now that we've learned about singular essential oils, let's delve a bit into making aromatherapy blends. Aromatherapists categorize essential oils into components or what are called "notes". As a musician, I like to think of it as notes of a chord.

Each essential oil is categorized as a top, middle or base note. Some oils can even have components of all three notes, but is usually categorized as a dominant single note.

Each blend should be comprised of the three main notes:

Top Note: The top note is the scent you notice first. It defines the blend and doesn't usually last long.

Middle Note: The middle note is sometimes referred to as the heart of the blend. It lasts about one to two hours.

Base or Bottom Note: The bottom note appears much later than the first two notes, sometimes hours or even a day later. It is the essential oil that gives the blend staying power and will linger long after the others have faded.

Let's begin by choosing five essential oils. Just pick five that you think will smell nice together and that you enjoy. Don't worry about top, middle and base notes right now.

For the next step, it's very helpful to have aromatherapy testing wands and your journal handy. If you don't have testing wands, you can cut small strips from white construction paper, creating your own. We're not all fancy pants here. Place one drop of each of your chosen essential oils on one wand together.

Grab your journal and start taking notes. What is your first impression of your blend? Does it make you feel any particular way? Relaxed? Uplifted? Does it remind you of a particular event from your past?

Let the essential oil blend evaporate and dry for about twenty minutes. If you need to, sniff some coffee grounds to clear your nose. Now, smell your aromatherapy testing wand again. Has the scent changed? Do you still smell all the original oils? Does it make you feel differently? What do you notice that has changed? Write all your impressions in your journal.

Now, look at the essential oils you've chosen. See what notes you have. A traditionally balanced blend will have two top, two middle and one bottom or base note.

Something else to consider is essential oil aroma strength. Each essential oil is distilled differently and each has it's own particular scent and strength. Some smell more potent than others, which can lead to them dominating your blend.

An easy way to test the balance of your blend is to take five aromatherapy testing wands and place a drop of each oil on an individual wand. Waft your aromatherapy testing wands in front of your nose, like a fan. Are you able to smell all of your essential oils? Do some stand out more than others? Are some very faint? Write your findings down in your journal. Add a drop to each aromatherapy strip that seems to be too light. This is your blend, so have fun! Keep track of the drops you add and to which strip.

There is no right or wrong. Once you've found your "perfect blend", write down your final formula in drops per essential oil. This will make it easier to add to recipes in the future.

Congratulations! You've created your first custom aromatherapy blend!

8

ESSENTIAL OIL DILUTION AND CONVERSIONS

This is the part of aromatherapy that is usually the most challenging. Conversions and dilutions. I'm going to try and make it easy. Conversions are just what they sound like; conversions from one system to another. Dilutions are the ratio of essential oils to carrier oils.

The first topic we'll talk about is conversions. You'll notice that most essential oil bottles are labeled in milliliters and most oils and other ingredients are listed in ounces. Here's a list of ounces converted to milliliters.

1/8 ounce is 3.75 milliliters
1/4 ounce is 7.5 milliliters
1/2 ounce is 15 milliliters
1 ounce is 30 milliliters
4 ounces is 120 milliliters
8 ounces is 237 milliliters
16 ounces is 473 milliliters

Although a one ounce bottle of essential oil is usually listed as 30 milliliters, it is technically 29.57 milliliters. It's rounded up to make it easier to work with.

Next, lets talk about ounces converted to drops. As a rule, there are about twenty drops of essential oils in 1 milliliter.

1/8 ounce is 75 drops
1/4 ounce is 150 drops
1/2 ounce is 300 drops
1 ounce is 600 drops

It's time to pull out your journal and write these conversions down. You'll be happy you did when you're in the middle of a recipe and need to do a quick conversion.

The second part of the conversation is dilutions. Essential oils are very strong and need to be diluted in a carrier oil before applying to the skin. Here's a simple chart of how much essential oil to add to a one ounce finished product or carrier oil.

1% Dilution
1 ounce = 30 ml = 600 drops of oil
1% of 600 drops is 6

Therefore, add six drops of essential oil to one ounce of a carrier oil for a one percent dilution.

2% Dilution
1 ounce = 30 ml = 600 drops of oil
2% of 600 drops is 12
Therefore, add twelve drops of essential oil to one ounce of carrier oil for a two percent dilution.

If you are using more than one essential oil, the drops are the total amount of drops you should add.   For example, for a one percent dilution using lavender and chamomile essential oils, you'd add a total of six drops of your essential oil blend to one ounce of a carrier oil, not twelve drops.

9

AROMATHERAPY AND CHILDREN

One thing to keep in mind when using essential oils in your home is that special care needs to be taken around children. Kids are not just mini adults. They're not only getting taller, their organs are still developing. Children's lungs are not fully developed until they're around three years old and their skin is more sensitive, among other things. Therefore, I don't recommend using essential oils on children until they are at least two years old. Even then, it's vital to talk to an experienced aromatherapist and your medical doctor to ensure the essential oils are suitable for your child.

Another thing to be very cautious of is the purity of your essential oils and carrier oils. It's even more important to use trusted, high quality ingredients on children less than ten years old.

There are different dilutions used for children, based upon their age and weight. As not all essential oils are suitable for children, it's important to follow guidelines and safety precautions set from an aromatherapist before using.

Here's a general guide of essential oils that are safe for children from two years to ten years old.

Basil
Bergamot
Blue Tansy
Catnip
Cedarwood
German Chamomile
Roman Chamomile
Citronella
Clary Sage
Copaiba Balsam
Coriander
Dill Weed
Fir Needle
Frankincense
Geranium
Ginger Root CO_2
Pink Grapefruit
Helichrysum
Jasmine Absolute
Juniper Berry
Lavender
Lavandin

Lemon
Mandarin
Marjoram
Neroli
Orange
Palmarosa
Patchouli
Petitgrain
Pine
Rosalina
Rose Absolute
Sandalwood
Spearmint
Spruce
Tangerine
Tea Tree
Vanilla 12%
Vetiver

For children two years old to six years old, I recommend a dilution of .25%. A dilution of .25% equals one drop of essential oil per four teaspoons of carrier oil. It may not seem like much, but as we know, essential oils are highly concentrated. That combined with the little ones size, make one drop perfect.

For children that are a bit older, six years to ten years old, I recommend a dilution of one percent. A one percent dilution is equal to 1 drop per 1 teaspoon of carrier oil. For more detailed instructions on one percent dilutions, please see the Dilution section of this book.

Here are a few suggestion of essential oils to use for kids issues:

Calming Oils
Blue Tansy
Clary Sage
Lavender
Sweet Orange
Neroli
Australian Sandalwood

Oils for Congestion
Frankincense
Juniper Berry
Cypress
Sweet Marjoram
Fir Needle
Pine

Sleepy Time Oils
Roman Chamomile
Clary Sage
Lavender
Rose Absolute
Coriander
Petitgrain

Cuts and Scrapes
Tea Tree
Lavender
Helichrysum
Juniper Berry

There are entire books devoted to using essential oils on children. I encourage you to delve further into this topic if you're going to incorporate essential oils into topical application for your children. Always remember, a little goes a long way and err on the side of caution for your precious children.

10

ESSENTIAL OILS
AND PREGNANCY

First of all, if you're reading this, you're probably expecting. Congratulations! What a wonderful and exciting time of your life. I understand it can also be a very stressful and anxious time. As you're trying to grow a beautiful baby, you can feel a bit out of sorts. Aromatherapy can help! Although there are some essential oils you want to avoid, you can safely incorporate aromatherapy into your life.

During pregnancy, I recommend a dilution of one percent. That is for essential oils that are deemed "safe" for you to use at all. A one percent dilution is equal to one drop of essential oil per one teaspoon of carrier oil.

There is a great deal of controversy about using essential oils and aromatherapy during pregnancy. The concern is the oils crossing the placenta. There have been no recorded cases of miscarriage or birth defect resulting from therapeutic application of essential oils during pregnancy. My advice is to follow your heart.

If you aren't comfortable using aromatherapy in the first trimester, then don't. You need to honor your body. If you were to use an essential oil to help with stress, and then were worried the whole time it was hurting your baby you'd override any calming effects. Plus we're trying to help you feel better, not add more stress. I encourage you to do research and consult with an experienced aromatherapist and your obstetrician.

The following is a list of essential oils that are commonly considered safe for use during pregnancy and nursing:

Bergamot
Cedarwood
German Chamomile
Roman Chamomile
Cypress
Fir Needle
Frankincense
Geranium
Ginger
Helichrysum
Juniper
Lavender
Lemon
Mandarin
Marjoram
Neroli
Patchouli
Petitgrain
Rose
Sandalwood
Sweet Orange
Tea Tree
Vetiver
Ylang Ylang

*Peppermint is a controversial oil. It is commonly considered safe to use in pregnancy, but is not recommended while breastfeeding

Most often during pregnancy, your sense of smell if heightened. Usually, citrus oils are the most comforting. The main benefit of using Aromatherapy while pregnant is the relief of tension and stress. There are ways an experienced aromatherapist can help, but it would require a consultation, as all mamas and babies are different.

A few common essential oil blends to help with conditions during pregnancy:

Morning Sickness
Petitgrain
Sweet Orange
Mandarin

Water Retention
Petitgrain
Geranium
Bitter Orange

Stretch Marks
Frankincense
Lavender
Rose
Roman Chamomile

11

LET'S GET DIFFUSING

We've spent some time learning about aromatherapy diffusers and diffusion blends, so now let's start filling your home with the beautiful scents of essential oils. Don't be afraid to experiment try your hand at making your own blend. The worst thing that will happen is you'll have to toss the water and oils and start again. I've included a few blends to get you started. Just add the drops to your diffuser and enjoy!

Calming Blends

Peace
10 drops of Lavender Essential Oil
6 drops of Chamomile Essential Oil

Relax
2 drops of Jasmine Essential Oil
2 drops of Lavender Essential Oil
15 drops of Vanilla Essential Oil

Unwind
2 drops of Lavender Essential Oil
2 drops of Sandalwood Essential Oil
1 drop of Chamomile Essential Oil

Energizing Blends

Cheer
6 drops Tangerine Essential Oil
2 drops Lemon Essential Oil
2 drops Grapefruit Essential Oil

Energy
2 drops Cinnamon Essential Oil
1 drop Rosemary Essential Oil
1 drop Peppermint Essential Oil

Uplift
1 drop Grapefruit Essential Oil
1 drop Peppermint Essential Oil
1 drop Lavender Essential Oil

Balancing Blends

Meditation
3 drops Patchouli Essential Oil
2 drops Clove Essential Oil
2 drops Sandalwood Essential Oil

Focus
3 drops Eucalyptus Globulus Oil
2 drops Sweet Orange Essential Oil
2 drops Peppermint Essential Oil

Clarity
2 drops Clary Sage Essential Oil
2 drops Rose Absolute Essential Oil
2 drops Geranium Essential Oil

Love is in the Air Blends

Bliss
2 drops Ylang Ylang Essential Oil
5 drops Rose Absolute Essential Oil

Passion
6 drops Jasmine Essential Oil
5 drops Geranium Essential Oil

Love
5 drops Geranium Essential Oil
3 drops Jasmine Absolute Essential Oil
1 drop Patchouli Essential Oil

Please follow the directions on your diffuser for setup and use. Essential Oils are highly concentrated and should be used with extreme care. Make sure to diffuse in a well ventilated area. Be careful not to diffuse on wooden furniture or delicate surfaces. Please keep all essential oils out of the reach of children and pets. Blends are suggested for adults only. Not for internal use. Always avoid contact with eyes and mucous membranes. Consult your healthcare practitioner before using if experiencing any health concerns, if you are pregnant or nursing.

12

AROMATHERAPY ON THE GO

Now, let's use all this knowledge and take aromatherapy with you! Always make sure you've followed the procedures for correct dilution before putting anything on your skin. For safe body application, test a bit on a small area of your skin. If you have any signs of redness, itching or irritation, discontinue use immediately. You can try to soothe the irritation with a bit of a carrier oil. If your spot test is a success, you can continue on to apply your blend to key areas of your body.

There are many areas on your body that you can apply essential oils to get the most therapeutic benefits. A few key areas we'll discuss are: the hairline by the temples, neck, behind your ears, the tops and soles of your feet, your neck and abdomen. You'll apply your aromatherapy to different areas of your body, depending on the support you need.

Headache and neck tension: apply diluted essential oils to the hairline by your temples (the heat from your body will move the oils to the temple area) and either the base of the head or forehead, depending on where your head or neck tension is

Overall well being: Apply diluted essential oils to the insides of your wrists and in the middle of your chest

Colds and congestion: Apply diluted essential oils to the soles of the feet and to the chest area. Also, try the recipe for Facial Steam in the Recipes section.

Stomachache and nausea: Apply diluted essential oils to the abdomen and gently massage in a circular motion

Muscle Pain: Apply diluted essential oils directly to the specific area of concern and gently massage into skin

For less specific use of aromatherapy, try taking a bath. It may sound simple, but a bath can change your life! Mix your essential oils with salts and soak in a warm bath for twenty minutes. Baths are wonderful for joint pain, muscle issues, stress, tension and insomnia.

Aromatherapy and massages go hand in hand. What better way to destress and rejuvenate than with a massage? Add some essential oils and you're on your way to pure bliss. Try adding twelve drops of your essential oil blend to one ounce of organic, unscented massage oil. Massage into the skin in small circular motions and watch your stress melt away.

In general, apply essential oils directly to the body for physical ailments and use inhalation therapy for emotional issues.

13

IT'S ALL IN THE PACKAGING

Now that you've learned about essential oils and how to blend them, it's time to talk about how to store them. Remember, essential oils are unstable, so they need to be stored in a cool, dark environment. They also are very concentrated, so any old plastic bottle won't do, you need to use glass. The plastic will just melt and your blend will be lost. Well made glass bottles are now available in a bunch of styles online that are specifically made for aromatherapy.

One of the first things you'll probably make is a room spray. To preserve your aromatherapy mists and sprays, use tinted glass bottles with fine mister tops. Some of the less expensive spray bottles tend to leak, so test your mist before tossing it in your purse. When filling your bottles, leave a little room at the top of the bottle to help with dripping.

Another type of bottle you can use for blends, is a glass bottle with a special carbonic top.

They're called Boston Rounds and are most commonly available in two colors, cobalt blue or amber. They work well for lotions and massage oils and any thinner liquid that uses a twist top.

The internet has made it much easier to have access to aromatherapy bottles. You can purchase the same kind of essential oil bottles your singular notes are packaged in. They're available in a bunch of sizes. I recommend starting with the 5 ml size for your blends. Look for the kind that comes with an orfice reducer. They are plastic tops that snap into the bottles and control the output of essential oils to just a drop at a time. Most single essential oil bottle come with them installed, so you probably already know what I mean. They'll save you more than once from cleaning up a spilled blend.

Glass roll on bottles are also a good choice to have on hand. You can blend your essential oils into a carrier oil, put it in the roll on bottle, snap on the top and take your personal perfume with you on the go. A quick tip, most of the tops snap in easily at first and then you need to snap them in further a second time to really seal the top. The plastic part should be flush with the glass on the side. If not, you may not have it sealed properly.

As far as storing your bath salts, you want to find a jar that has a tight lid that won't let any moisture in. My favorite jars are tinted mason jars. I always keep them on hand in a few sizes because I find I use them for everything: bath salts, sugar scrubs, thicker body butters, you name it. They're economical and really work well! You can even dress them up with ribbon and fabric for gift giving. Yard sales and vintage shops are great places to find beautiful bottles, too. Just make sure the tops close tightly

As you can see, there are lots of choices for storage for your aromatherapy creations. Just follow the few simple rules that I mentioned, and the sky is the limit.

14

AROMATHERAPY RECIPES

Here are a few tried an true recipes that will get you started. As you become more comfortable in your blending abilities, feel free to change out the essential oils to create different blends.

Aromatherapy Body Spray

2 ounce tinted, light mist, glass spray bottle
1/2 teaspoon vodka
1/2 teaspoon aloe vera gel
1/2 teaspoon glycerin
1/2 teaspoon witch hazel
distilled water
10-20 drops of essential oils

How to Make:

Add vodka, aloe vera gel, glycerin and witch hazel to the 2 ounce tinted spray bottle. Fill the rest with distilled water. Shake very well. Add your essential oils and shake again. Lightly mist over your head.

*Make sure to be careful when spraying your mist. Avoid spraying on furniture or over food and drink.

Relaxing Spa Bath Salts

Ingredients:

4 cups Epsom Salts
2 cups Fine Sea Salts
10 drops of Sweet Orange Essential Oil
15 drops of Lavender Essential Oil

How to Make:

Mix salts together well in a bowl. Slowly add in essential oils. Package in a tightly sealed glass jar. Fill your bathtub with warm water. Once tub is full, put 1 cup of salts in the water. Swirl and enjoy!

Sea Salt Body Scrub

Ingredients:

1 cup of Fine Sea Salt
1/2 cup of Sweet Almond or Fractionated
Coconut Oil
10 drops of Lavender Essential Oil

How to Make:

Mix all ingredients together in a small bowl.
Place in a sealed glass container.

Massage gently into the skin and rinse off with
warm water. Be careful, your tub may be
slippery.

Whipped Coconut Oil Body Butter

Ingredients:

1 cup virgin coconut oil
1 teaspoon vitamin E oil
20 drops of essential oil

How to Make:

Put all the ingredients into the mixing bowl of a stand mixer.

Mix on high speed with a wire whisk for 7-8 minutes or until whipped into a light, frosting consistency

Spoon the body butter into a glass jar and seal tightly. Coconut Oil can liquify in very warm temperatures, so place in the refrigerator during hot spells.

A little bit will go a long way. Apply a small amount to your body after your shower for soft, moisturized skin.

Stress Relief Massage Oil

Ingredients:

1/4 cup jojoba oil for carrier oil
5 drops of Sweet Orange Essential Oil
5 drops Frankincense Essential Oil
1 drop Jasmine Essential Oil

How to Make:

Combine all the ingredients in a dark glass jar with a lotion dispenser cap.

Wait at least 24 hours before using to let the blend settle. Store your Stress Relief Massage Oil in a cool, dark place. Best if used within three months. This recipe can be doubled.

Steam Treatment for Coughs and Colds

Ingredients:

4 cups of boiling water
1 drop of Frankincense Essential Oil
2 drops of Ravensara Essential Oil
a large towel

How to Make:

Boil the water in a tea kettle or pot on the stove. Transfer the boiling water to a heat safe bowl and add the essential oils. Drape a towel over your head, close your eyes and lower your face toward the bowl.

Trap the steam with the towel around the edges of the bowl, so you get maximum benefits of the essential oil blend rising from the boiling water. Breathe deeply for ten minutes.

You can repeat the steam treatment again, later in the day until your cough and cold subsides.

All Purpose Cleaning Spray

Ingredients:
2 Cups of Distilled Water
2 Cups of White Vinegar
1 teaspoon of unscented natural dish soap
(I use Seventh Generation)
30 drops of Lemon Essential Oil
20 drops of Tea Tree Essential Oil

How to Make:

Mix all the ingredients in a quart sized, tinted glass spray bottle. Shake well to combine. Spray lightly on non porous surfaces. Wipe off with a clean cloth.

This spray works wonders on countertops, toilets, sinks and anywhere else that needs freshening.

15

THE END IS JUST
THE BEGINNING

Thank you so much for joining me on this fascinating journey. In the chapters that have preceded, I have shared a lot of information with you about aromatherapy and essential oils. I hope you have found it easy to read and implement into your life. My biggest wish is to have inspired you to look at an alternative way of healing through the use of essential oils and simple, natural ingredients.

I have created "The Essential Art of Aromatherapy" to serve as an introduction, and I encourage you to pick up the torch and carry on from here. There are vast amounts of information about aromatherapy and essential oil recipes available today and I hope that you will continue on your path. Even after studying for the better part of thirty years, I still learn something every day. Take a deep breath and enjoy all the benefits of aromatherapy!

16

QUICK TIPS

Build your Aromatherapy collection by purchasing quality, undiluted, pure essential oils, not perfume or fragrance oils.

Do not apply pure essential oils directly to your skin without mixing with a carrier oil. I strongly recommend never ingesting essential oils.

Store your essential oils in tinted amber or cobalt blue glass bottles. A cool, dark place will keep them fresh longer. Do not use rubber glass dropper tops or plastic bottles, as they'll disintegrate from the concentrated oils.

Always err on the side of caution. Safety is very important when blending and using potent essential oils. Follow dilution guidelines and patch test if trying a new oil for the first time. Refer to the list of essential oils for special considerations, like health concerns, using on children and pregnancy. If you have any questions at all, consult your physician and an experienced aromatherapist prior to using.

Do continue your studies of aromatherapy but reading the suggested resources and talking with experienced aromatherapists. Beware of blog posts and information from aromatherapy beginners.

Common Carrier Oils:
Fractionated Coconut Oil, Sweet Almond Oil, Jojoba, Avocado, Hemp Seed Oil

Relaxing Essential Oils:
Lavender, Chamomile, Bergamot, Vetiver, Ylang Ylang, Frankincense, Rose, Lemon, Geranium, Marjoram

Energizing Essential Oils:
Grapefruit, Ginger, Juniper Berry, Lemongrass, Rosemary, Clary Sage, Spearmint, Bergamot, Peppermint

Cleansing Essential Oils:
Tea Tree, Lemon, Wild Orange, Lavender, Eucalyptus, Peppermint, Cinnamon Leaf, Rosemary

Cold and Flu Fighters:
Lavender, Eucalyptus, Tea Tree, Cypress, Lemon, Lemongrass, White Thyme, Peppermint, Sage and Rosemary

Most importantly, have fun! You've begun a wonderful journey!

17

RESOURCES

Essential Oils and Supplies:

twig leaf flower
www.twigleafflower.com
I am very partial to this one, because it's my company. I offer a full organic vegan aromatherapy collection, including diffusion blends. My recipes reflect the wisdom of generations of women in my family and the knowledge I've acquired from amazing teachers in the more than twenty five years I've practiced in the wellness industry.

Plant Therapy
www.planttherapy.com
This is a wonderful essential oil company that has partnered with Robert Tisserand, one of the pioneers in aromatherapy. He's written countless books and is considered the authority on the practice of aromatherapy. Plant Therapy offers a complete line of pure, organic essential oils and has an informative blog for further study.

Mountain Rose Herbs
www.mountainroseherbs.com
Rosemary Gladstar is a trailblazer in modern herbalism. She has taught thousands of herbalists throughout the world and is one of my dearest teachers. Years ago, Rosemary started a small herbal business in California to provide class supplies for her students. When she moved to Vermont, Rose Madrone took over the herbal business and Mountain Rose Herbals was born. They are amazing stewards to the environment, respect the beauty of organic practices and offer an extensive line of essential oils, carriers, bottles and containers.

Bulk Apothecary
www.bulkapothecary.com
Bulk Apothecary is a great resource for quality, fair priced containers and product bases.

Books:

The Complete Book of Essential Oils and Aromatherapy by Valerie Ann Worwood

Back to Eden by Jethro Kloss

The Art of Aromatherapy: The Healing and Beautifying Properties of the Essential Oils of Flowers and Herbs by Robert B. Tisserand

Advanced Aromatherapy-The Science of Essential Oil Therapy by Kurt Schnaubelt, Ph.D.

Essential Oil Safety: A Guide for Health Care Professionals by Robert Tisserand and Rodney Young

Aromatherapy for the Healthy Child by Valerie Ann Worwood

Aromatherapy- A Complete Guide to the Healing Art by Kathi Keville and Mindy Green

The Healing Intelligence of Essential Oils-The Science of Advanced Aromatherapy by Kurt Schnaubelt, Ph. D.

The Essential Oils Handbook by Jennie Harding

Organic Body Care Recipes by Stephanie Tousles

The Practice of Aromatherapy by Jean Valnet

Gattefosse's Aromatherapy: The First Book on Aromatherapy by Rene-Maurice Gattefosse

Essential Living by Andrea Butje

The Encyclopedia of Essential Oils: The Complete Guide to the Use of Aromatic Oils in

Aromatherapy, Herbalism, Health and Wellbeing by Julia Lawless

18

SPECIAL PRECAUTIONS

Please note that this listing is not exhaustive. As we've discussed, you should always consult your physician and an experienced aromatherapist before using any essential oils if you are experiencing any underlying health concerns or are pregnant or nursing.

Prolonged inhalation of concentrated essential oils can cause headaches, dizziness and nausea. Please avoid the listed essential oils if you experience any of the following conditions.

Cancer:
Aniseed, Basil, Bay Laurel, Clove, Cinnamon, Fennel, Ho Leaf, Nutmeg and Star Anise

Estrogen Dependent Cancer:
Aniseed, Citronella, Eucalyptus, Fennel, Lemongrass, Star Anise and Verbena

Skin Cancer:
Bergamot and all sun sensitizing oils

Epilepsy and Seizures:
Fennel, Hyssop, Nutmeg, Rosemary and Sage

High Blood Pressure:
Hyssop, Rosemary, Sage and Thyme

Pregnancy:
See chapter regarding essential oils and pregnancy

Skin Irritants:
A few essential oils may cause skin irritation in some individuals. I recommend patch testing before using any oils. You should never use any essential oil undiluted on the skin without professional advice, especially Basil, Black Pepper, Clove, Cinnamon, Ginger, Lemon, Lemongrass, Oregano, Peppermint and Pine.

Skin Sensitizers:
These oils have a higher tendency to create a sensitivity reaction: Peru Balsam, Basil, Cinnamon, Bay Laurel, Lemon, Lemongrass, Melissa, Peppermint, Thyme and Tea Tree Oil.

Sun Sensitizers:
Essential Oils can cause sensitivity to the sun, especially those from the citrus family. Avoid ultraviolet light and sun exposure after applying: Bergamot, Bitter Orange, Grapefruit, Lemon, Lime, Orange, Mandarin and Tangerine.

ABOUT THE AUTHOR

Rebecca Nicely is an aromatherapist and herbalist from Dallas, PA. She has a passion for reconnecting people to the incredible wonder of nature and loves creating simple rituals to enhance lives. She's a professional member of National Holistic Aromatherapy Association and owns her own organic vegan aromatherapy and herbal company, **twig leaf flower**. Rebecca has been blessed to have worked and studied with leaders in the holistic wellness industry for over twenty five years and has practiced healing modalities for most of her life. She believes her greatest accomplishment is the love she brings into the world by continuing the legacy of her herbalist grandmothers.

You can reach Rebecca at the following links

Website
http://www.twigleafflower.com/

Email
rebecca@twigleafflower.com

Blog
https://twigleafflower.wordpress.com

Facebook
https://www.facebook.com/twigleafflower

Instagram
https://www.instagram.com/twigleafflower/

Twitter
https://twitter.com/twigleafflower

naha page
https://www.naha.org